The Keto Vegetarian Way of Living

Be Healthy with Delicious

Keto Vegetarian Recipes

Ricardo Abagnale

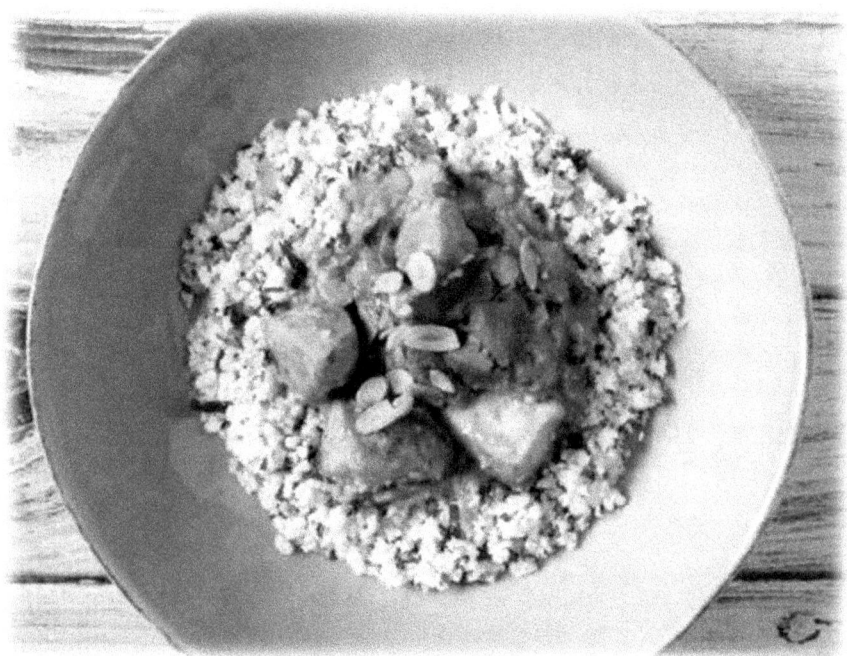

by reading this document, the reader agrees that under no circumstances is the author responsible for any losses, direct or indirect, which are incurred as a result of the use of information contained within this document, including, but not limited to, — errors, omissions, or inaccuracies.

Table of Contents

INTRODUCTION

The Ketogenic diet is truly life changing. The diet improves your overall health and helps you lose the extra weight in a matter of days. The diet will show its multiple benefits even from the beginning and it will become your new lifestyle really soon.

As soon as you embrace the Ketogenic diet, you will start to live a completely new life.

On the other hand, the vegetarian diet is such a healthy dietary option you can choose when trying to live healthy and also lose some weight.

The collection we bring to you today is actually a combination between the Ketogenic and vegetarian diets. You get to discover some amazing Ketogenic vegetarian dishes you can prepare in the comfort of your own home. All the dishes you found here follow both the Ketogenic and the vegetarian rules, they all taste delicious and rich and they are all easy to make.

We can assure you that such a combo is hard to find. So, start a keto diet with a vegetarian "touch" today. It will be both useful and fun!

So, what are you still waiting for? Get started with the Ketogenic diet and learn how to prepare the best and most flavored Ketogenic vegetarian dishes. Enjoy them all!

BREAKFAST

Vegetarian Keto Breakfast Frittata

Preparation time: 10 minutes
Cooking time: 5 minutes
Servings: 4

Ingredients:

- 4 organic eggs
- ¼ teaspoon sea salt
- 1 avocado, peeled, sliced
- 2-ounces cheddar cheese, shredded
- 10 olives, pitted
- teaspoon herb de Provence
- 2 tablespoons olive oil
- 2 tablespoons butter

Nutritional Values (Per Serving):

- Calories: 346
- Fat: 32.8 g

- Carbohydrates: 5.5 g
- Sugar: 0.7 g
- Protein: 10.2 g
- Cholesterol: 194 mg

Directions:

1. In a mixing bowl, add herb de Provence, eggs, olives, sea salt and whisk until frothy. Melt the butter in a pan over high heat. Add avocado slices to pan and cook until lightly golden brown. Remove from pan and set aside.
2. Pour the egg mixture into the pan and sprinkle cheese on top over the top of egg mixture. Cover pan with lid and cook for 3 minutes. Flip over to other side and cook for another 2 minutes.
3. Transfer the frittata to serving plate and top with avocado slices. Enjoy!

Creamy Cheese Soufflés

Preparation time: 10 minutes

Cooking time: 25 minutes

Servings: 8

Nutritional Values (Per Serving):

- Calories: 214
- Fat: 17.9 g
- Carbohydrates: 1.6 g
- Sugar: 0.5 g
- Protein: 11.6 g
- Cholesterol: 168 mg

Ingredients:

- 6 organic eggs, separated
- 1 teaspoon salt
- ½ cup almond flour
- 1 teaspoon mustard, ground
- ½ teaspoon pepper
- ½ teaspoon xanthan gum
- ¼ teaspoon cayenne pepper

- ¾ cup heavy cream
- 2 cups cheddar cheese, shredded
- tablespoons chives, fresh, chopped
- ¼ teaspoon cream of tartar

Directions:

1. Preheat your oven to 350°Fahrenheit. Spray 8 ramekins with cooking spray and place them onto a cookie sheet.
2. In a mixing bowl, whisk together pepper, mustard, cayenne, xanthan gum, salt and almond flour. Slowly add in the cream and mix until well combined.
3. Whisk your egg yolks, cheese, chives until well blended. In another mixing bowl, beat the egg whites with the cream of tartar until stiff peaks are formed. Gently fold egg whites into the cheese and almond flour mixture. Pour the mixture into prepared ramekins.
4. Bake in preheated oven for 25 minutes or until your soufflés are lightly golden brown. Serve and enjoy!

Keto Zucchini Fritters

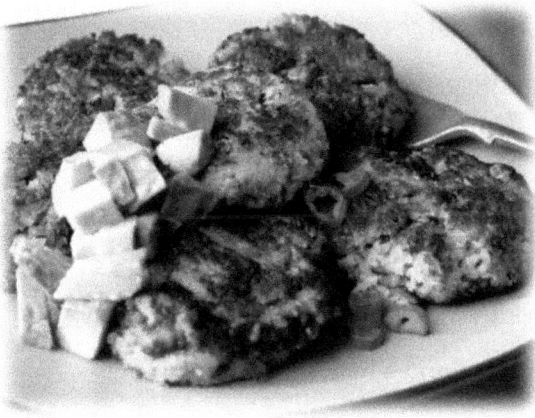

Preparation time: 25 minutes

Cooking time: 6 minutes

Servings: 8

Nutritional Values (Per Serving):

- Calories: 81
- Fat: 6 g
- Carbohydrates: 5 g
- Sugar: 0 g
- Protein: 5 g
- Cholesterol: 58 mg

Ingredients:

- lb. zucchini, grated and squeezed
- 1 teaspoon salt
- 2 organic eggs
- 1 ½ ounces onion, minced
- 1 teaspoon lemon pepper
- ½ teaspoon baking powder
- ½ cup almond flour
- ¼ coconut flour
- ¼ cup Parmesan cheese, grated

Directions:

1. Add your zucchini, eggs, and onion in a mixing bowl and mix until well combined.
2. Add all the remaining ingredients into another mixing bowl, and stir well. Add your dry ingredients to the zucchini mixture and mix well.
3. Pour enough oil into the pan to cover the bottom surface of it. Heat the oil over medium-high heat. Once the oil becomes hot, pour ¼ cup zucchini batter into pan and cook for 3 minutes then flip and cook the other side for another 3 minutes.
4. Place your fried zucchini fritters on a paper towel to soak up the excess oil. Serve and enjoy!

MAINS

Grilled Veggie Mix

Preparation time: 10 minutes

Cooking time: 30 minutes

Servings: 4

Nutritional Values (Per Serving):

- Calories 120
- Fat 1
- Fiber 3
- Carbs 9
- Protein 2

Ingredients:

- 1 pound cherry tomatoes, halved
- 2 eggplants, roughly cubed

- 2 cups radishes, halved
- 2 green bell peppers, halved, deseeded
- 1 teaspoon chili powder
- 1 teaspoon rosemary, dried
- 1/4 cup balsamic vinegar
- Salt and black pepper to the taste
- 2 tablespoons olive oil
- 1 tablespoon basil, chopped

Directions:

1. In a bowl, combine the tomatoes with the eggplants and the other ingredients except the basil and toss well.
2. Arrange the veggies on your preheated grill and cook over medium heat for 15 minutes on each side.
3. Divide the veggies between plates, sprinkle the basil on top and serve.

Vinegar Cucumber, Olives and Shallots Salad

Preparation time: 10 minutes

Cooking time: 0 minutes

Servings: 4

Nutritional Values (Per Serving):

- calories 120
- fat 3
- fiber 2
- carbs 5
- protein 10

Ingredients:

- 1 pound cucumbers, sliced
- 1 cup black olives, pitted and sliced
- 3 tablespoons shallots, chopped

- ¼ cup balsamic vinegar
- 1 tablespoon dill, chopped
- A pinch of salt and black pepper
- 3 tablespoons avocado oil

Directions:

1. In a bowl, mix the cucumbers with the olives, shallots and the other ingredients, toss well, divide between plates and serve.

Tomato and Peppers Pancakes

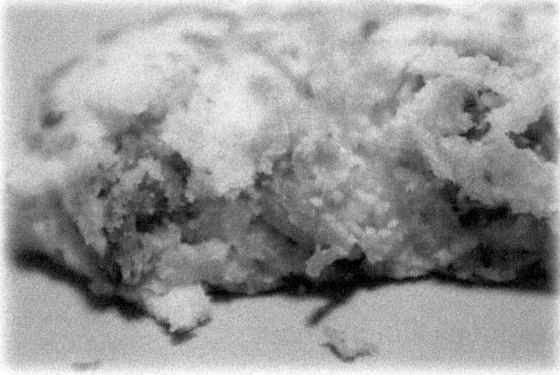

Preparation time: 10 minutes

Cooking time: 10 minutes

Servings: 4

Nutritional Values (Per Serving):

- Calories 70
- Fat 2
- Fiber 3
- Carbs 10
- Protein 4

Ingredients:

- 3 scallions, chopped
- 1 pound tomatoes, crushed
- 1 red bell pepper, chopped
- 1 green bell pepper, chopped
- Salt and black pepper to the taste
- 1 teaspoon coriander, ground
- 2 tablespoons almond flour
- 2 tablespoons flaxseed mixed with 3 tablespoons water
- 3 tablespoons coconut oil, melted

Directions:

1. In a bowl, combine the tomatoes with the peppers and the other ingredients except 1 tablespoon oil and stir really well.
2. Heat up a pan with the remaining oil over medium heat, add ¼ of the batter, spread into the pan, cook for 3 minutes on each side and transfer to a plate.
3. Repeat this with the rest of the batter, transfer all pancakes to a platter and serve.

Greens and Vinaigrette

Preparation time: 10 minutes

Cooking time: 0 minutes

Servings: 4

Nutritional Values (Per Serving):

- Calories 112
- Fat 9
- Fiber 2
- Carbs 6
- Protein 2

Ingredients:

- 1 cup baby kale
- 1 cup baby arugula
- 1 cup romaine lettuce
- 2 tomatoes, cubed
- 1 cucumber, cubed

- 3 tablespoons lime juice
- 1/3 cup olive oil
- 1 tablespoon balsamic vinegar
- Salt and black pepper to the taste

Directions:

1. In a bowl, combine the oil with the vinegar, lime juice, salt and pepper and whisk well.
2. In another bowl, combine the greens with the vinaigrette, toss and serve right away.

Mushroom and Mustard Greens Mix

Preparation time: 10 minutes

Cooking time: 20 minutes

Servings: 4

Nutritional Values (Per Serving):

- Calories 76
- Fat 1
- Fiber 2
- Carbs 3
- Protein 3

Ingredients:

- 1 pound white mushrooms, halved
- 2 cups mustard greens
- 1 tablespoon lime juice

- 3 scallions, chopped
- 2 tablespoons olive oil
- 1 teaspoon sweet paprika
- 1 teaspoon rosemary, dried
- 2 bunches parsley, chopped
- 3 garlic cloves, minced
- Salt and black pepper to the taste

Directions:

1. Heat up a pan with the oil over medium heat, add the scallions, paprika, garlic and parsley and sauté for 5 minutes.
2. Add the mushrooms and the other ingredients, toss, cook over medium heat for 15 minutes, divide between plates and serve.

Mustard Greens and Kale Mix

Preparation time: 10 minutes

Cooking time: 10 minutes

Servings: 4

Nutritional Values (Per Serving):

- Calories 200
- Fat 4
- Fiber 8
- Carbs 16
- Protein 7

Ingredients:

- 1 pound mustard greens
- ½ pound kale, torn
- 2 celery stalks, chopped
- 2 tablespoons avocado oil
- 1 cup tomatoes, cubed

- 2 avocados, peeled, pitted and cubed
- 1 cup coconut cream
- 2 tablespoons lemon juice
- 2 garlic cloves minced
- 2 tablespoons parsley, chopped
- A pinch of salt and black pepper

Directions:

1. Heat up a pan with the oil over medium heat, add the mustard greens, kale, celery and the other ingredients, toss, cook for 10 minutes, divide between plates and serve warm.

Zucchini Fries and Sauce

Preparation time: 10 minutes

Cooking time: 25 minutes

Servings: 4

Nutritional Values (Per Serving):

- calories 140
- fat 5
- fiber 2
- carbs 20
- protein 6

Ingredients:

- 1 pound zucchinis, cut into fries
- 2 tablespoons olive oil
- ½ teaspoon rosemary, dried
- 3 scallions, chopped
- 2 teaspoons smoked paprika

- A pinch of sea salt and black pepper
- 1 cup coconut cream
- 1 tablespoon balsamic vinegar
- ½ teaspoon garlic powder
- 2 tablespoons cilantro, chopped

Directions:

1. Arrange the zucchini fries on a baking sheet lined with parchment paper, add half of the oil, paprika, garlic powder, salt and pepper, toss and bake in the oven at 425 degrees F for 12 minutes.

2. Heat up a pan with the rest of the oil over medium heat, add the scallions and sauté for 3 minutes.

3. Add the cream and the remaining ingredients, toss, and cook over medium heat for 10 minutes more.

4. Divide the zucchini fries between plates, drizzle the sauce all over and serve.

Chard and Garlic Sauce

Preparation time: 10 minutes

Cooking time: 15 minutes

Servings: 4

Nutritional Values (Per Serving):

- Calories 374
- Fat 34.2
- Fiber 6.7
- Carbs 15.4
- Protein 9

Ingredients:

- ½ cup walnuts, chopped
- 4 cups red chard, torn
- 3 tablespoons olive oil
- Juice of 1 lime
- 1 celery stalks, chopped

- 1 cup coconut cream
- 4 garlic cloves, minced
- 1 tablespoon balsamic vinegar
- 2/3 cup scallions, chopped
- A pinch of sea salt and black pepper

Directions:

1. Heat up a pan with the oil over medium heat, add the scallions, garlic and the celery and sauté for 5 minutes.
2. Add the chard and the other ingredients, toss, cook over medium heat for 10 minutes more, divide between plates and serve.

Mushroom and Spinach Mix

Preparation time: 10 minutes

Cooking time: 15 minutes

Servings: 4

Nutritional Values (Per Serving)

- Calories 116
- Fat 11.3
- Fiber 1.1
- Carbs 3.5
- Protein 2.5

Ingredients:

- 1 cup white mushrooms, sliced
- 3 cups baby spinach
- 2 tablespoons olive oil

- Salt and black pepper to the taste
- 2 tablespoons garlic, minced
- 2 tablespoons pine nuts, toasted
- 1 tablespoon walnuts, chopped

Directions:

1. Heat up a pan with the oil over medium heat, add the garlic, pine nuts and the walnuts and cook for 5 minutes.
2. Add the mushrooms and the other ingredients, toss, cook over medium heat for 10 minutes, divide between plates and serve.

Garlic Cauliflower Rice

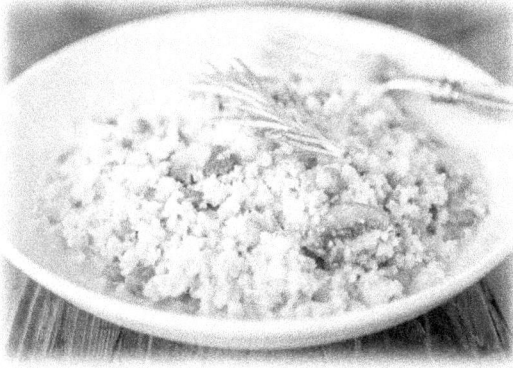

Preparation time: 10 minutes

Cooking time: 20 minutes

Servings: 4

Nutritional Values (Per Serving):

- Calories 142
- Fat 6.1
- Fiber 1.2
- Carbs 3
- Protein 1.2

Ingredients:

- 2 cups cauliflower rice
- 2 tablespoons almonds, chopped
- 1 tablespoon olive oil
- 2 green onions, chopped
- 4 garlic cloves, minced
- 3 tablespoons chives, chopped
- ½ cup vegetable stock

Directions:

1. Heat up a pan with the oil over medium heat, add the garlic and green onions and sauté for 5 minutes.
2. Add the cauliflower rice and the other ingredients, toss, cook over medium heat for 15 minutes, divide between plates and serve.

Grapes and Tomato Salad

Preparation time: 10 minutes

Cooking time: 0 minutes

Servings: 4

Nutritional Values (Per Serving):

- Calories 140
- Fat 4
- Fiber 6
- Carbs 3.4
- Protein 4

Ingredients:

- 2 cups green grapes, halved
- 1 pound cherry tomatoes, halved
- 2 tablespoons olive oil
- 4 spring onions, chopped
- 1 teaspoon cumin, ground

- 1 teaspoon rosemary, dried
- 1 tablespoon balsamic vinegar
- 1 tablespoon chives, chopped

Directions:

1. In a bowl, combine the grapes with the tomatoes and the other ingredients, toss and serve as a side salad.

Tomato and Walnuts Vinaigrette

Preparation time: 10 minutes

Cooking time: 0 minutes

Serving: 4

Nutritional Values (Per Serving):

- Calories 160
- Fat 12
- Fiber 4
- Carbs 6
- Protein 4

Ingredients:

- 1 pound cherry tomatoes, halved
- 1 tablespoon walnuts, chopped
- 1 tablespoon balsamic vinegar

- 1 garlic clove, minced
- 1 teaspoon lemon juice
- 2 teaspoons smoked paprika
- ¼ teaspoon coriander, ground
- Salt and black pepper to the taste
- 1 tablespoon parsley, chopped

Directions:

1. In a bowl, combine the tomatoes with the walnuts and the other ingredients, toss well, and serve as a side dish.

Creamy Eggplant Mix

Preparation time: 10 minutes

Cooking time: 15 minutes

Servings: 4

Nutritional Values (Per Serving):

- Calories 142
- Fat 7
- Fiber 4
- Carbs 5
- Protein 3

Ingredients:

- 1 pound eggplants, roughly cubed
- 2 scallions, chopped
- 2 tablespoons avocado oil
- 2 teaspoons garlic, minced

- ½ cup coconut cream
- 2 teaspoons chili paste

Directions:

1. Heat up a pan with the oil over medium heat, add the scallions and the garlic and sauté for 2 minutes.
2. Add the eggplants and the other ingredients, toss, cook over medium heat for 13 minutes more, divide between plates and serve as a side dish.

Chives Kale and Tomato

Preparation time: 10 minutes

Cooking time: 20 minutes

Servings: 4

Nutritional Values (Per Serving):

- Calories 128
- Fat 2.3
- Fiber 1
- Carbs 3.3
- Protein 4

Ingredients:

- 1 pound kale, torn
- ½ pound tomatoes, cut into wedges
- 2 tablespoons avocado oil
- 1 teaspoon chili powder
- 1 teaspoon garam masala

- Salt and black pepper to the taste
- ¼ teaspoon coriander, ground
- A pinch of cayenne pepper
- 1 teaspoon mustard powder
- ¼ cup chives, chopped

Directions:

1. In a roasting pan, combine the kale with the tomatoes and the other ingredients, toss and bake at 380 degrees F for 20 minutes.
2. Divide the mix between plates and serve as a side dish.

Miso Spaghetti Squash

Preparation time: 5 minutes

Cooking time: 40 minutes

Servings: 4

Nutritional Values (Per Serving):

- Calories: 117
- Fat: 2g
- Protein: 3g
- Carbohydrates: 25g
- Fiber: 0g
- Sugar: 0g
- Sodium: 218mg

Ingredients:

- 1 3-pound spaghetti squash
- 1 tablespoon hot water
- 1 tablespoon unseasoned rice vinegar
- 1 tablespoon white miso

Directions:

1. Preheat the oven to 400°F. Line a rimmed baking sheet with parchment paper. Halve the squash lengthwise and place, cut-side down, on the prepared baking sheet.

2. Bake for 35 to 40 minutes, until tender. Cool until the squash is easy to handle. With a fork, scrape out the flesh, which will be stringy, like spaghetti. Transfer to a large bowl. In a small bowl, combine the hot water, vinegar, and miso with a whisk or fork. Pour over the squash. Gently toss with tongs to coat the squash. Divide the squash evenly among 4 single-serving containers. Let cool before sealing the lids.

Braised Cabbage and Apples

Preparation time: 5 minutes

Cooking time: 25 minutes

Servings: 6

Ingredients:

- 2 tablespoons olive oil
- 1 small head red cabbage, shredded
- 1 small head savoy cabbage, shredded
- 1 Granny Smith apple
- 1 red cooking apple, such as Rome or Gala
- 2 tablespoons sugar
- 1 cup water
- 1/4 cup cider vinegar
- Salt and freshly ground black pepper

Directions:

1. In a large saucepan, heat the oil over medium heat. Add the shredded red and savoy cabbage, cover, and cook until slightly wilted, 5 minutes.

2. Core the apples and cut them into 1/4-inch dice. Add the apples to the cabbage, along with the sugar, water, vinegar, and salt and pepper to taste. Reduce heat to low, cover, and simmer until the cabbage and apples are tender, stirring frequently, about 20 minutes. Serve immediately.

Marsala Carrots

Preparation time: 5 minutes

Cooking time: 20 minutes

Servings: 4

Ingredients:

- 2 tablespoons vegan margarine
- 1 pound carrots, cut diagonally into 1/4-inch slices
- Salt and freshly ground black pepper
- 1/2 cup Marsala
- 1/4 cup water
- 1/4 cup chopped fresh parsley, for garnish

Directions:

1. In a large skillet, melt the margarine over medium heat. Add the carrots and toss well to coat evenly with the margarine. Cover and cook, stirring occasionally, for 5 minutes.

2. Season with salt and pepper to taste, tossing to coat. Add the Marsala and water. Reduce heat to low, cover, and simmer until the carrots are tender, about 15 minutes.
3. Uncover and cook over medium-high heat until the liquid is reduced into a syrupy sauce, stirring to prevent burning.
4. Transfer to a serving bowl and sprinkle with parsley. Serve immediately.

Garlic and Herb Zoodles

Preparation time: 10 minutes

Cooking time: 2 minutes

Servings: 4

Nutritional Values (Per Serving):

- Calories: 44
- Fat: 2g
- Protein: 3g
- Carbohydrates: 7g
- Fiber: 2g
- Sugar: 3g
- Sodium: 20mg

Ingredients:

- 1 teaspoon extra-virgin olive oil or 2 tablespoons vegetable broth
- 1 teaspoon minced garlic (about 1 clove)

- 4 medium zucchini, spiralized
- ½ teaspoon dried basil
- ½ teaspoon dried oregano
- ¼ to ½ teaspoon red pepper flakes, to taste
- ¼ teaspoon salt (optional
- ¼ teaspoon freshly ground black pepper

Directions:

1. In a large skillet over medium-high heat, heat the olive oil.
2. Add the garlic, zucchini, basil, oregano, red pepper flakes, salt (if using), and black pepper. Sauté for 1 to 2 minutes, until barely tender. Divide the zoodles evenly among 4 storage containers. Let cool before sealing the lids.

Ratatouille (Pressure cooker)

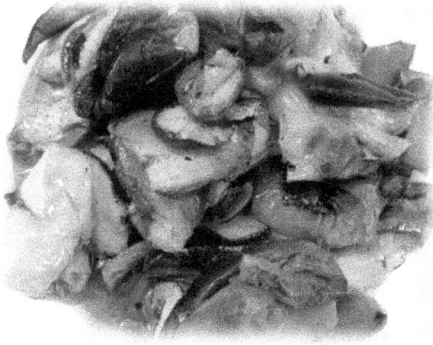

Preparation time: 15 minutes

Servings: 4-6

Nutritional Values (Per Serving):

- Calories: 101
- Total fat: 2g
- Protein: 4g
- Sodium: 304mg
- Fiber: 7g

Ingredients:

- 1 onion, diced
- 4 garlic cloves, minced
- 1 to 2 teaspoons olive oil
- 1 cup water
- 3 or 4 tomatoes, diced
- 1 eggplant, cubed
- 1 or 2 bell peppers, any color, seeded and chopped
- 1½ tablespoons dried herbes de Provence (or any mixture of dried basil, oregano, thyme, marjoram, and rosemary)
- ½ teaspoon salt
- Freshly ground black pepper

Directions:

1. On your electric pressure cooker, select Sauté. Add the onion, garlic, and olive oil. Cook for 4 to 5 minutes, stirring occasionally, until the onion is softened. Add the water, tomatoes, eggplant, bell peppers, and herbes de Provence. Cancel Sauté.

2. High pressure for 6 minutes. Close and lock the lid and ensure the pressure valve is sealed, then select High Pressure and set the time for 6 minutes.

3. Pressure Release. Once the cook time is complete, let the pressure release naturally, about 20 minutes. Once all the pressure has released, carefully unlock and remove the lid. Let cool for a few minutes, then season with salt and pepper.

Cream of Artichoke Soup

Preparation time: 10 minutes

Cooking time: 20 minutes

Servings: 4

Ingredients:

- 1 tablespoon olive oil
- 2 medium shallots, chopped
- 2 10-ouncepackages frozen artichoke hearts, thawed
- 3 cups vegetable broth (homemade, store-bought, or water)
- 1 teaspoon fresh lemon juice
- Salt
- 1/3 cup almond butter
- 1/8 teaspoon ground cayenne
- 1 cup plain unsweetened soy milk

- 1 tablespoon snipped fresh chives, for garnish
- 2 tablespoons sliced toasted almonds, for garnish

Directions:

1. In a large soup pot, heat the oil over medium heat. Add the shallots, cover, and cook until softened. Uncover and stir in the artichoke hearts, broth, lemon juice, and salt to taste. Bring to a boil, then reduce heat to low and simmer, uncovered, until the artichokes are tender, about 20 minutes.

2. Add the almond butter and cayenne to the artichoke mixture. Puree in a high-speed blender or food processor, in batches if necessary, and return to the pot. Stir in the soy milk and taste, adjusting seasonings if necessary. Simmer the soup over medium heat until hot, about 5 minutes.

3. Ladle into bowls, sprinkle with chives and almonds, and serve.

Pomegranate-Infused Lentil and Chickpea Stew

Preparation time: 5 minutes

Cooking time: 55 minutes

Servings: 4

Ingredients:

- ¾ cup brown lentils, picked over, rinsed, and drained
- 2 tablespoons olive oil
- ½ cup chopped green onions
- 2 teaspoons minced fresh ginger
- ¾ cup long-grain brown rice
- ½ cup dried apricots, quartered
- ¼ cup golden raisins
- ¼ teaspoon ground allspice
- ¼ teaspoon ground cumin
- ¼ teaspoon ground cayenne
- 1 teaspoon turmeric
- Salt and freshly ground black pepper

- 1/3 cup pomegranate molasses, homemade or store-bought
- 3 cups water
- 1 1/2 cups cooked or 1 15.5-ouncecan chickpeas, drained and rinsed
- 1/4 cup minced fresh cilantro or parsley

Directions:

1. Soak the lentils in a medium bowl of hot water for 45 minutes. Drain and set aside.
2. In a large saucepan, heat the oil over medium heat. Add the green onions, ginger, soaked lentils, rice, apricots, raisins, allspice, cumin, cayenne, turmeric, and salt and pepper to taste. Cook, stirring, for 1 minute.
3. Add the pomegranate molasses and water and bring to a boil. Reduce heat to low. Cover and simmer until the lentils and rice are tender, about 40 minutes.
4. Stir in the chickpeas and cilantro. Simmer, uncovered, for 15 minutes, to heat through and allow the flavors to blend. Serve immediately.

Rice and Pea Soup

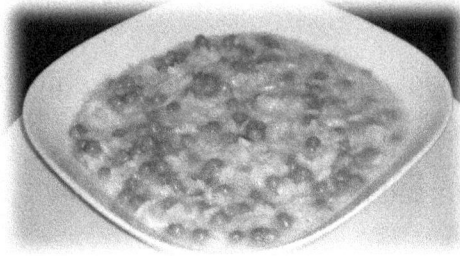

Preparation time: 5 minutes

Cooking time: 45 minutes

Servings: 4

Ingredients:

- 2 tablespoons olive oil
- 1 medium onion, minced
- 2 garlic cloves minced
- 1 cup Arborio rice
- 6 cups vegetable broth, homemade, store-bought, or water
- Salt and freshly ground black pepper

- 1 16-ouncebag frozen petite green peas
- 1⁄4 cup chopped fresh flat-leaf parsley

Directions:

1. In a large soup pot, heat the oil over medium heat. Add the onion and garlic, cover, and cook until softened about 5 minutes.
2. Uncover and add the rice, broth, and salt and pepper to taste. Bring to a boil, then reduce heat to low. Cover and simmer until the rice begins to soften, about 30 minutes.
3. Stir in the peas and cook, uncovered, for 15 to 20 minutes longer. Stir in the parsley and serve.

Ethiopian Cabbage, Carrot, and Potato Stew

Preparation time: 10 minutes

Cooking time: 20 minutes

Servings: 6

Ingredients:

- 3 russet potatoes, peeled and cut into ½-inch cubes
- 2 tablespoons olive oil
- 6 carrots, peeled, halved lengthwise, and cut into ½-inch slices
- 1 onion, chopped
- 4 garlic cloves, minced
- 1 tablespoon ground turmeric
- 1 teaspoon ground cumin
- 1 teaspoon ground ginger
- 1½ teaspoons sea salt

- 1½ cups low-sodium vegetable broth, divided
- 4 cups shredded or thinly sliced green cabbage

Directions:

1. Bring a large pot of water to a boil over medium-high heat.
2. Add the potatoes and cook for 10 minutes, or until fork-tender. Drain and set aside. While the potatoes are cooking, heat the oil in a large skillet over medium-high heat. Add the carrots and onion and sauté for 5 minutes. Add the garlic, turmeric, cumin, ginger, and salt and sauté for 1 additional minute, until fragrant. Add the cooked potatoes and 1 cup of broth to the skillet, bring to a boil, and reduce to a simmer. Scatter the cabbage on top of the potatoes. Cover and simmer for 3 minutes.
3. Mix the cabbage into the potatoes, add the remaining ½ cup of broth, cover, and simmer for 5 more minutes, or until the cabbage is wilted and tender. Stir the cabbage from time to time while cooking to incorporate it with the other ingredients as it continues to wilt.

Coconut Tofu Zucchini Bake

Preparation time: 40 minutes

Serving: 4

Nutritional Values (Per Serving):

- Calories: 492
- Total Fat:26.8 g
- Saturated Fat: 12.6g
- Total Carbs: 14g
- Dietary Fiber:4g
- Sugar: 8g, Protein: 50g
- Sodium: 1668mg

Ingredients:

- 1 tbsp butter
- 1 cup green beans, chopped

- 1 bunch asparagus, trimmed and cut into 1-inch pieces
- 2 tbsp arrowroot starch
- 2 cups coconut milk
- 4 medium zucchinis, spiralized
- 1 cup grated parmesan cheese
- 1 (15 oz) firm tofu, pressed and sliced
- Salt and black pepper to taste

Directions:

1. Preheat the oven to 380 F.
2. Melt the butter in a medium skillet and sauté the green beans and asparagus until softened, about 5 minutes. Set aside.
3. In a medium saucepan, mix the arrowroot starch with the coconut milk. Bring to a boil over medium heat with frequent stirring until thickened, 3 minutes. Stir in half of the parmesan cheese until melted.
4. Mix in the green beans, asparagus, zucchinis and tofu. Season with salt and black pepper.
5. Transfer the mixture to a baking dish and cover the top with the remaining parmesan cheese.

6. Bake in the oven until the cheese melts and golden on top, 20 minutes.

7. Remove the food from the oven and serve warm.

Not-Tuna Salad

Preparation time: 5 minutes

Cooking time: 0 minutes

Servings: 4

Nutritional Values (Per Serving):

- Calories: 214
- Fat: 6g
- Protein: 9g
- Carbohydrates: 35g
- Fiber: 8g
- Sugar: 1g
- Sodium: 765mg

Ingredients:

- 1 (15.5-ouncecan chickpeas, drained and rinsed
- 1 (14-ouncecan hearts of palm, drained and chopped
- ½ cup chopped yellow or white onion
- ½ cup diced celery
- ¼ cup vegan mayonnaise, plus more if needed
- ½ teaspoon salt
- ¼ teaspoon freshly ground black pepper

Directions:

1   In a medium bowl, use a potato masher or fork to roughly mash the chickpeas until chunky and "shredded." Add the hearts of palm, onion, celery, vegan mayonnaise, salt, and pepper.

2   Combine and add more mayonnaise, if necessary, for a creamy texture. Into each of 4 single-serving containers, place ¾ cup of salad. Seal the lids.

Dazzling Vegetable Salad

Preparation time: 15 minutes

Cooking time: 0 minutes

Servings: 4

Ingredients:

- 1 medium carrot, shredded
- 1 cup finely shredded red cabbage
- 1 cup ripe grape or cherry tomatoes, halved
- 1 medium yellow bell pepper, cut into matchsticks
- 1½ cups cooked or 1 (15.5-ouncecan chickpeas, rinsed and drained
- ¼ cup halved pitted kalamata olives
- ripe Hass avocado, pitted, peeled, and cut into ½-inch dice
- ¼ cup olive oil
- 1½ tablespoons fresh lemon juice
- ½ teaspoon salt

- ⅛ teaspoon freshly ground black pepper
- Pinch sugar (optional)

Directions:

1. In a large bowl, combine the watercress, carrot, cabbage, tomatoes, bell pepper, chickpeas, olives, and avocado and set aside.
2. In a small bowl, combine the oil, lemon juice, salt, black pepper, and sugar. Blend well and add to the salad. Toss gently to combine and serve.

Red Bean and Corn Salad

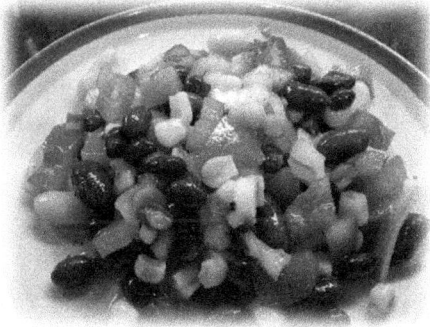

Preparation time: 15 minutes

Cooking time: 0 minutes

Servings: 4

Nutritional Values (Per Serving):

- Calories: 303
- Fat: 9g
- Protein: 14g
- Carbohydrates: 45g
- Fiber: 15g
- Sugar: 6g
- Sodium: 654mg

Ingredients:

- ¼ cup Cashew Cream or other salad dressing
- 1 teaspoon chili powder
- (14.5-ouncecans kidney beans, rinsed and drained
- cups frozen corn, thawed, or 2 cups canned corn, drained
- 1 cup cooked farro, barley, or rice (optional)
- 8 cups chopped romaine lettuce

Directions:

1. Line up 4 wide-mouth glass quart jars.
2. In a small bowl, whisk the cream and chili powder. Pour 1 tablespoon of cream into each jar. In each jar, add ¾ cup kidney beans, ½ cup corn, ¼ cup cooked farro (if using), and 2 cups romaine, punching it down to fit it into the jar. Close the lids tightly.

Mango and Snow Pea Salad

Preparation time: 15 minutes

Cooking time: 0 minutes

Servings: 4

Ingredients:

- 1⁄2 teaspoon minced garlic
- 1⁄2 teaspoon grated fresh ginger
- 1⁄4 cup creamy peanut butter
- 1 tablespoon plus 1 teaspoon light brown sugar
- 1⁄4 teaspoon crushed red pepper
- tablespoons rice vinegar
- 3 tablespoons water
- tablespoon soy sauce
- cups snow peas, trimmed and lightly blanched
- 1⁄2 cup chopped unsalted roasted peanuts, for garnish
- 1 medium cucumber, peeled, halved lengthwise, and seeded
- 3 cups shredded romaine lettuce

- 2 ripe mangos, peeled, pitted, cut into ½-inch dice
- 1 large carrot, shredded

Directions:

1.   In a small bowl, combine the garlic, ginger, peanut butter, sugar, and crushed red pepper. Stir in the vinegar, water, and soy sauce. Taste, adjusting seasonings, if necessary, and set aside.

2.   Cut the snow peas diagonally into a thin matchsticks and place in a large bowl. Add the mangos and carrot. Cut the cucumber into ¼-inch slices and add to the bowl.

3.   Pour the dressing onto the salad and toss gently to combine. Spoon the salad onto a bed of shredded lettuce, sprinkle with peanuts, and serve.

Savory Seed Crackers

Preparation time: 5 minutes

Cooking time: 50 minutes

Servings: 20 crackers

Nutrition (5 crackers):

- Calories: 339
- Fat: 29g
- Protein: 14g
- Carbohydrates: 17g
- Fiber: 8g
- Sugar: 1g
- Sodium: 96mg

Ingredients:

- ¾ cup pumpkin seeds (pepitas)
- ½ cup sunflower seeds
- ½ cup sesame seeds
- ¼ cup chia seeds
- 1 teaspoon minced garlic (about 1 clove)
- 1 teaspoon tamari or soy sauce
- 1 teaspoon vegan Worcestershire sauce
- ½ teaspoon ground cayenne pepper
- ½ teaspoon dried oregano
- ½ cup water

Directions:

1. Preheat the oven to 325°F.
2. Line a rimmed baking sheet with parchment paper.
3. In a large bowl, combine the pumpkin seeds, sunflower seeds, sesame seeds, chia seeds, garlic, tamari, Worcestershire sauce, cayenne, oregano, and water.
4. Transfer to the prepared baking sheet, spreading out to all sides.
5. Bake for 25 minutes. Remove the pan from the oven, and flip the seed "dough" over so the wet side is up.

Bake for another 20 to 25 minutes, until the sides are browned.

6. Cool completely before breaking up into 20 pieces. Divide evenly among 4 glass jars and close tightly with lids.

Tomato and Basil Bruschetta

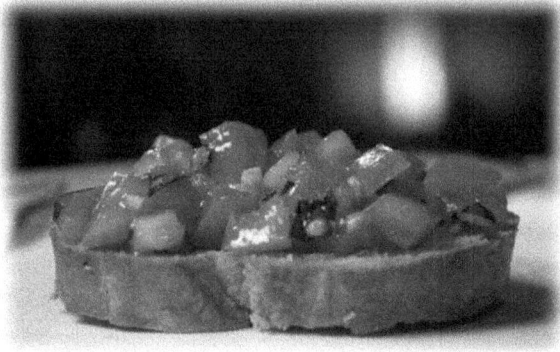

Preparation time: 10 minutes

Cooking time: 6 minutes

Servings: 12 bruschetta

Ingredients:

- 3 tomatoes, chopped
- ¼ cup chopped fresh basil
- 1 tablespoon olive oil pinch of sea salt
- 1 baguette, cut into 12 slices
- 1 garlic clove, sliced in half

Directions:

1. In a small bowl, combine the tomatoes, basil, olive oil, and salt and stir to mix. Set aside. Preheat the oven to 425°F.
2. Place the baguette slices in a single layer on a baking sheet and toast in the oven until brown, about 6 minutes.
3. Flip the bread slices over once during cooking. Remove from the oven and rub the bread on both sides with the sliced clove of garlic.
4. Top with the tomato-basil mixture and serve immediately.

Refried Bean and Salsa Quesadillas

Preparation time: 5 minutes

Cooking time: 6 minutes

Servings: 4 quesadillas

Ingredients:

- 1 tablespoon canola oil, plus more for frying
- 1½ cups cooked or 1 (15.5-ouncecan pinto beans, drained and mashed
- 1 teaspoon chili powder
- 4 (10-inchwhole-wheat flour tortillas
- 1 cup tomato salsa, homemade or store-bought
- ½ cup minced red onion (optional

Directions:

1. In a medium saucepan, heat the oil over medium heat. Add the mashed beans and chili powder and cook, stirring, until hot, about 5 minutes. Set aside.

2. To assemble, place 1 tortilla on a work surface and spoon about 1/4 cup of the beans across the bottom half. Top the beans with the salsa and onion, if using. Fold top half of the tortilla over the filling and press slightly.

3. In large skillet heat a thin layer of oil over medium heat. Place folded quesadillas, 1 or 2 at a time, into the hot skillet and heat until hot, turning once, about 1 minute per side.

4. Cut quesadillas into 3 or 4 wedges and arrange on plates. Serve immediately.

Tempeh Tantrum Burgers

Preparation time: 15 minutes

Cooking time: 0 minutes

Servings: 4 burgers

Ingredients:

- 8 ounces tempeh, cut into 1⁄2-inch dice
- 3⁄4 cup chopped onion
- 2 garlic cloves, chopped
- 3⁄4 cup chopped walnuts
- 1⁄2 cup old-fashioned or quick-cooking oats
- 1 tablespoon minced fresh parsley
- 1⁄2 teaspoon dried oregano
- 1⁄2 teaspoon dried thyme
- 1⁄2 teaspoon salt
- 1⁄4 teaspoon freshly ground black pepper
- 3 tablespoons olive oil
- Dijon mustard

- 4 whole grain burger rolls
- Sliced red onion, tomato, lettuce, and avocado

Directions:

1. In a medium saucepan of simmering water, cook the tempeh for 30 minutes. Drain and set aside to cool.
2. In a food processor, combine the onion and garlic and process until minced. Add the cooled tempeh, the walnuts, oats, parsley, oregano, thyme, salt, and pepper. Process until well blended. Shape the mixture into 4 equal patties.
3. In a large skillet, heat the oil over medium heat. Add the burgers and cook until cooked thoroughly and browned on both sides, about 7 minutes per side.
4. Spread desired amount of mustard onto each half of the rolls and layer each roll with lettuce, tomato, red onion, and avocado, as desired. Serve immediately.

Sesame- Wonton Crisps

Preparation time: 10 minutes

Cooking time: 10 minutes

Servings: 12 crisps

Ingredients:

- 12 Vegan Wonton Wrappers
- 2 tablespoons toasted sesame oil
- 12 shiitake mushrooms, lightly rinsed, patted dry, stemmed, and cut into 1⁄4-inch slices
- 4 snow peas, trimmed and cut crosswise into thin slivers
- 1 teaspoon soy sauce
- 1 tablespoon fresh lime juice
- 1⁄2 teaspoon brown sugar
- 1 medium carrot, shredded
- Toasted sesame seeds or black sesame seeds, if available

Directions:

1. Preheat the oven to 350°F. Lightly oil a baking sheet and set aside. Brush the wonton wrappers with 1 tablespoon of the sesame oil and arrange on the baking sheet. Bake until golden brown and crisp, about 5 minutes. Set aside to cool. (Alternately, you can tuck the wonton wrappers into mini-muffin tins to create cups for the filling. Brush with sesame oil and bake them until crisp.

2. In a large skillet, heat the extra olive oil over medium heat. Add the mushrooms and cook until softened, 3 to 5 minutes. Stir in the snow peas and the soy sauce and cook 30 seconds. Set aside to cool.

3. In a large bowl, combine the lime juice, sugar, and remaining 1 tablespoon sesame oil. Stir in the carrot and cooled shiitake mixture. Top each wonton crisp with a spoonful of the shiitake mixture. Sprinkle with sesame seeds and arrange on a platter to serve.

Cocoa Muffins

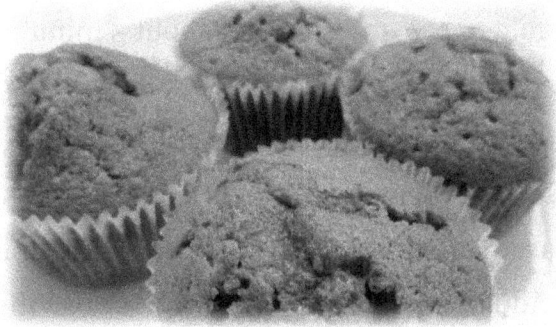

Preparation time: 10 minutes

Cooking time: 25 minutes

Servings: 6

Nutritional Values (Per Serving):

- calories 344
- fat 35.1
- fiber 3.4

- carbs 8.3
- protein 4.5

Ingredients:

- ½ cup coconut oil, melted
- 3 tablespoons stevia
- 1 cup almond flour
- ¼ cup cocoa powder
- 3 tablespoons flaxseed mixed with 4 tablespoons water
- ¼ teaspoon vanilla extract
- 1 teaspoon baking powder
- Cooking spray

Directions:

1. In bowl, combine the coconut oil with the stevia, the flour and the other ingredients except the cooking spray and whisk well.
2. Grease a muffin pan with the cooking spray, divide the muffin mix in each mould, bake at 370 degrees F for 25 minutes, cool down and serve.

Melon Coconut Mousse

Preparation time: 10 minutes

Cooking time: 0 minutes

Servings: 6

Nutritional Values (Per Serving):

- Calories 219
- Fat 21.1
- Fiber 0.9
- Carbs 7
- Protein 1.4

Ingredients:

- 2 cups coconut cream
- 1 teaspoon vanilla extract
- 1 tablespoon stevia
- 1 cup melon, peeled and chopped

Directions:

In a blender, combine the melon with the cream and the other ingredients, pulse well, divide into bowls and serve cold.

Chia and Strawberries Mix

Preparation time: 10 minutes

Cooking time: 0 minutes

Servings: 4

Nutritional Values (Per Serving):

- Calories 265
- Fat 6.3
- Fiber 2
- Carbs 4
- Protein 6

Ingredients:

- 1 cup strawberries, halved
- 2 tablespoons chia seeds
- ¼ cup coconut milk
- 1 tablespoon stevia

Directions:

1. In a bowl, combine the berries with the chia seeds, the milk and stevia and whisk well.
2. Divide the mix into bowls and serve cold.

Watermelon Mousse

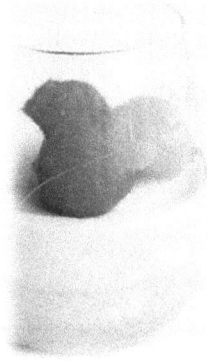

Preparation time: 10 minutes

Cooking time: 0 minutes

Servings: 4

Nutritional Values (Per Serving):

- Calories 332
- Fat 31.4
- Fiber 0.5
- Carbs 9.2
- Protein 5.5

Ingredients:

- 1 cup coconut cream
- 1 tablespoon lemon juice
- 1 tablespoon stevia
- 2 cups watermelon, peeled and cubed

Directions:

1. In a blender, combine the watermelon with the cream, the lemon juice and stevia, pulse well, divide into bowls and serve cold.

Fruit Salad

Preparation time: 2 hours

Cooking time: 0 minutes

Servings: 4

Nutritional Values (Per Serving):

- Calories 243
- Fat 22
- Fiber 0
- Carbs 6.2
- Protein 4

Ingredients:

- 2 avocados, peeled, pitted and cubed
- ½ cup blackberries
- ½ cup strawberries, halved
- ½ cup pineapple, peeled and cubed
- ¼ teaspoon vanilla extract

- 2 tablespoons stevia
- Juice of 1 lime

Directions:

1. In a bowl, combine the avocados with the berries and the other ingredients, toss and keep in the fridge for 2 hours before serving.

Chia Bars

Preparation time: 10 minutes

Cooking time: 20 minutes

Servings: 6

Nutritional Values (Per Serving):

- Calories 220
- Fat 2
- Fiber 0.5
- Carbs 2
- Protein 4

Ingredients:

- 1 cup coconut oil, melted
- ½ teaspoon baking soda
- 3 tablespoons chia seeds
- 2 tablespoons stevia
- 1 cup coconut cream

- 3 tablespoons flaxseed mixed with 4 tablespoons water

Directions:

1. In a bowl, combine the coconut oil with the cream, the chia seeds and the other ingredients, whisk well, pour everything into a square baking dish, introduce in the oven at 370 degrees F and bake for 20 minutes.
2. Cool down, slice into squares and serve.

Fruits Stew

Preparation time: 10 minutes

Cooking time: 10 minutes

Servings: 4

Nutritional Values (Per Serving):

- Calories 178
- Fat 4.4
- Fiber 2
- Carbs 3
- Protein 5

Ingredients:

- 1 avocado, peeled, pitted and sliced
- 1 cup plums, stoned and halved
- 2 cups water
- 2 teaspoons vanilla extract

- 1 tablespoon lemon juice
- 2 tablespoons stevia

Directions:

1. In a pan, combine the avocado with the plums, water and the other ingredients, bring to a simmer and cook over medium heat for 10 minutes.
2. Divide the mix into bowls and serve cold.

Avocado and Rhubarb Salad

Preparation time: 10 minutes

Cooking time: 0 minutes

Servings: 4

Nutritional Values (Per Serving):

- Calories 140
- Fat 2
- Fiber 2
- Carbs 4
- Protein 4

Ingredients:

- 1 tablespoon stevia
- 1 cup rhubarb, sliced and boiled
- 2 avocados, peeled, pitted and sliced
- 1 teaspoon vanilla extract
- Juice of 1 lime

Directions:

1. In a bowl, combine the rhubarb with the avocado and the other ingredients, toss and serve.

Plums and Nuts Bowls

Preparation time: 5 minutes

Cooking time: 0 minutes

Servings: 2

Nutritional Values (Per Serving):

- Calories 400
- Fat 23
- Fiber 4
- Carbs 6
- Protein 7

Ingredients:

- 2 tablespoons stevia
- 1 cup walnuts, chopped
- 1 cup plums, pitted and halved
- 1 teaspoon vanilla extract

Directions:

1. In a bowl, mix the plums with the walnuts and the other ingredients, toss, divide into 2 bowls and serve cold.

Crunchy Cauliflower Bites

Preparation time: 10 minutes

Cooking time: 20 minutes

Servings: 8

Nutritions:

- Calories: 81
- Sugar: 1.3 g
- Fat: 2.4 g
- Carbohydrates: 10.7 g
- Cholesterol: 42 mg
- Protein: 4.3 g

Ingredients:

- 2 eggs, organic, beaten
- 1 tablespoon Parmesan cheese, grated

- ½ head cauliflower, cut into florets
- 1 cup breadcrumbs
- Pepper and salt to taste

Directions:

1. Preheat your oven to 395°Fahrenheit. Spray baking dish with cooking spray and set aside. In a shallow dish combine the cheese, breadcrumbs, pepper, and salt. Dip the cauliflower florets in beaten egg then roll in breadcrumb mixture. Place coated cauliflower florets onto prepared baking dish. Bake in preheated oven for 20 minutes. Serve hot and enjoy!

Crispy Zucchini Fries

Preparation time: 10 minutes

Cooking time: 25 minutes

Servings: 4

Nutritions:

- Calories: 149
- Sugar: 2.6 g
- Cholesterol: 11 mg
- Fat: 8.1 g
- Carbohydrates: 13.6 g
- Proteins: 6 g

Ingredients:

- 1 medium zucchini
- 4 tablespoons almond meal
- 4 tablespoons light ranch dressing
- 3 tablespoons Franks hot sauce

- 2 teaspoons Italian seasoning
- ½ cup breadcrumbs
- 2 tablespoons Parmesan cheese, grated

Directions:

1. Preheat oven to 395° Fahrenheit. Spray a baking dish with cooking spray and set aside. Wash zucchini and cut into fries' size pieces. Place almond meal in a flat dish. Take another flat dish and mix the breadcrumbs, Italian seasoning, and cheese on it. In a bowl combine the hot sauce and ranch dressing. Roll zucchini pieces in the almond meal then dip in sauce mixture and finally coat with breadcrumb mixture. Place coated zucchini on prepared baking dish. Bake in preheated oven for 25 minutes. Flip zucchini fries once halfway through. Serve and enjoy!

Crispy Kale Chips

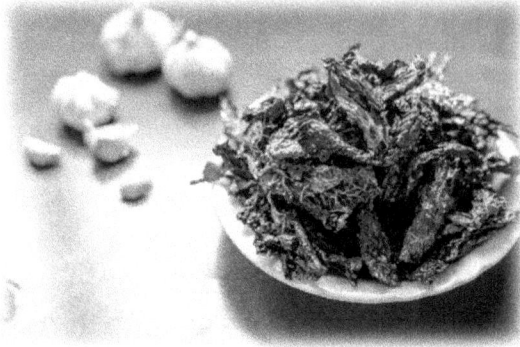

Preparation time: 10 minutes

Cooking time: 12 minutes

Servings: 2

Nutritions:

- Calories: 55
- Carbohydrates: 5.2 g
- Fat: 2.3 g
- Sugar: 0 g
- Cholesterol: 0 mg
- Protein: 2 g

Ingredients:

- 1 cup kale, fresh
- 2 teaspoons garlic seasoning
- 2 teaspoons sesame seeds, toasted

Directions:

1. Preheat your oven to 325° Fahrenheit. Spray baking dish with cooking spray and set aside. Wash kale and pat dry with paper towel. Cut the kale and tear into pieces and place in a baking dish. Spray kale with cooking spray. Sprinkle sesame seeds and seasoning over the kale. Bake in preheated oven for 12 minutes. Serve and enjoy.

Vegan Chocolate Bars

Preparation time: 10 minutes

Cooking time: 1 hour

Servings: 3

Nutritions:

- Calories 182
- Fat 15 g
- Carbohydrates 12.3 g
- Sugar 11 g
- Protein 3.2 g
- Cholesterol 0 mg

Ingredients:

- 2 lbs. summer squash, cut into 1-inch pieces
- 1/8 tsp pepper
- 1/8 tsp garlic powder
- 3 tbsp olive oil

- 1 large lemon juice
- 1/8 tsp paprika Pepper
- Salt

Directions:

1. Preheat the oven to 400 F/ 204 C.
2. Spray a baking tray with cooking spray.
3. Place squash pieces onto the prepared baking tray and drizzle with olive oil.
4. Season with paprika, pepper, and garlic powder.
5. Squeeze lemon juice over the squash and bake in preheated oven for 50-60 minutes.
6. Serve hot and enjoy.

Brown Fat Bombs

Preparation time: 7 minutes

Cooking time: 30 minutes

Servings: 2

Nutritions:

- Calories 266
- Fat 24.7
- Fiber 8.3
- Carbs 12.6
- Protein 3.7

Ingredients:

- 1 teaspoon vanilla extract
- 1/3 teaspoon instant coffee
- 1 tablespoon liquid stevia
- 2 tablespoon cocoa powder

- ¾ teaspoon salt
- 1/3 cup coconut butter

Directions:

1. Take the mixing bowl and combine together vanilla extract, liquid stevia, and instant coffee.
2. Add salt and melted butter.
3. After this, add cocoa powder and mix up the ingredients until you get a soft and smooth texture.
4. Transfer the mixture into the ice cube molds and flatten the surface gently.
5. Place the ice cube molds in the freezer and let them stay there for 30 minutes.

www.ingramcontent.com/pod-product-compliance
Lightning Source LLC
Chambersburg PA
CBHW050749030426
42336CB00012B/1735